Fernando Antônio Ramos Schramm Neto

Pocket guide: Exanthematous diseases in childhood

Fernando Antônio Ramos Schramm Neto

Pocket guide: Exanthematous diseases in childhood

The main features in simple, dynamic language!

ScienciaScripts

Imprint

Any brand names and product names mentioned in this book are subject to trademark, brand or patent protection and are trademarks or registered trademarks of their respective holders. The use of brand names, product names, common names, trade names, product descriptions etc. even without a particular marking in this work is in no way to be construed to mean that such names may be regarded as unrestricted in respect of trademark and brand protection legislation and could thus be used by anyone.

Cover image: www.ingimage.com

This book is a translation from the original published under ISBN 978-620-6-76076-4.

Publisher:
Sciencia Scripts
is a trademark of
Dodo Books Indian Ocean Ltd. and OmniScriptum S.R.L publishing group

120 High Road, East Finchley, London, N2 9ED, United Kingdom
Str. Armeneasca 28/1, office 1, Chisinau MD-2012, Republic of Moldova, Europe
Printed at: see last page
ISBN: 978-620-8-14451-7

CONTENTS

INTRODUCTION

Dear readers,

We are delighted to present this book, dedicated to the main exanthematous diseases in childhood. These diseases, which manifest themselves with skin rashes, are common in children's lives and can cause a great deal of concern. Our aim is to provide clear and useful information so that you, parents, educators and health professionals, can better understand these conditions and care for children more calmly and confidently.

Here you will find detailed chapters on diseases such as chickenpox, measles, rubella and others. Each chapter covers the symptoms, forms of transmission, prevention measures and available treatments. Everything has been written in a simple and straightforward manner, so that even those without a medical background can understand and apply the information in their daily lives.

More than just presenting technical data, we want to talk to you about the concerns and doubts that arise when a child has a rash. We know that seeing a sick child is distressing, and we hope that this book can be a source of comfort and clarification. Our intention is to demystify these diseases, making it easier to recognize them and deal with them appropriately.

We invite you to dive into this reading, which has been prepared with great care and dedication. We hope that each page brings you valuable knowledge and helps to alleviate the uncertainties that these diseases can cause. By the end of this book, we hope that you will feel more prepared and secure in caring for your children, knowing how to identify the warning signs and when to seek medical help.

We thank you for trusting in our work and hope that this book will be an important ally in promoting children's health and well-being. Happy reading and may this journey be filled with learning and peace of mind.

CHAPTER 1. CHICKENPOX

1.1 DEFINITION

Chickenpox, better known as chickenpox, is a common disease, especially in children. It is characterized by rashes on the skin that cause itching and can turn into small blisters filled with fluid. Chickenpox is highly contagious and spreads easily from one person to another.

The history of chickenpox goes back many centuries, but it was at the end of the 19th century that doctors began to understand it better. Before that, it was often confused with other skin diseases. With the advance of science, it was discovered that chickenpox is caused by a virus and not bacteria, as many initially thought.

The main characteristics of chickenpox include a mild fever, tiredness, loss of appetite and, of course, the famous rash. These rashes usually start on the face, chest and back, quickly spreading all over the body. They go through several phases: they start as small red spots, develop into fluid-filled blisters and finally form scabs before disappearing.

The etiological agent of chickenpox is the varicella-zoster virus (VZV), a member of the herpesvirus family. This virus is responsible for both chickenpox and shingles (also known as mumps), which can occur later in life. Initial infection with the virus causes chickenpox, while reactivation of the latent virus in the body can result in shingles.

The varicella-zoster virus is transmitted through direct contact with the rash or through the air when an infected person coughs or sneezes. It is therefore very easy to contract chickenpox if you have not been vaccinated or have not had the disease before. The good news is that most people acquire immunity after infection or vaccination.

Finally, the prevention of chickenpox is possible through the vaccine, which is highly effective and usually administered in two doses. Vaccination not only protects the individual, but also helps prevent the spread of the disease in the community. So understanding chickenpox, its characteristics and how it is transmitted can help you take steps to protect the health of children and everyone around you.

1.2 EPIDEMIOLOGY

Chickenpox is a common disease that mainly affects children, but can occur at any age. Before the introduction of the vaccine, almost all children had chickenpox at some point. Globally, vaccination against chickenpox has significantly reduced the number of cases. In countries where vaccination is widely practiced, the incidence of chickenpox has fallen dramatically, making the disease much less common than it was in the past.

In Brazil, vaccination against chickenpox was introduced into the national immunization schedule in 2013. Since then, the prevalence of the disease has dropped significantly. Recent data shows that, thanks to vaccination, the number of cases of chickenpox has steadily decreased, also reducing hospitalizations and serious complications associated with the disease. Before vaccination, there were hundreds of thousands of cases a year, but now the numbers are much lower, reflecting the success of vaccination campaigns.

However, chickenpox is still a concern in areas where the vaccine is not widely accessible. In many developing countries, the disease remains a common cause of doctor visits and hospitalizations for children. The World Health Organization (WHO) and other public health organizations continue to work to improve access to the vaccine worldwide, with the aim of further reducing the global incidence of chickenpox and protecting the health of children everywhere.

1.3 PHYSIOPATHOLOGY

When a person is infected with VZV, the virus enters the body via the respiratory tract or through direct contact with the skin lesions of an infected person.

Once in the body, the virus multiplies in the cells of the upper respiratory tract and then spreads through the blood to the skin. This spread is what causes the characteristic chickenpox rash. The lesions start as small red spots, develop into fluid-filled blisters, and finally form scabs before disappearing. This cycle usually lasts 5 to 10 days.

The incubation period for chickenpox, i.e. the time between exposure to the virus and the appearance of symptoms, ranges from 10 to 21 days. During this period, the virus replicates silently inside the body. Chickenpox is most contagious one to two days before the rash appears until all the blisters have turned into scabs.

Transmission of the varicella-zoster virus occurs mainly through the air, via respiratory droplets expelled when the infected person coughs or sneezes. It can also occur through direct contact with skin lesions. Due to its high contagiousness, it is easy to understand how chickenpox can spread rapidly in environments such as schools and nurseries.

To prevent chickenpox, the vaccine is the most effective tool. Vaccination not only protects the individual, but also reduces the spread of the virus in the community. The chickenpox vaccine is usually given in two doses, one at 12-15 months of age and another between 4 and 6 years. People who have not been vaccinated and have not had the disease can also be vaccinated at a later date.

In addition to vaccination, hygiene measures, such as frequent hand washing and avoiding contact with infected people, are important to prevent transmission of the virus. In cases where chickenpox develops, isolating the infected individual helps to minimize the spread of the disease.

Despite being a common disease, chickenpox can lead to serious complications, especially in people with weakened immune systems, pregnant women and newborn babies. Complications can include secondary bacterial skin infections, pneumonia and encephalitis. This is why prevention through vaccination is so crucial.

Understanding the pathophysiology and ways of preventing chickenpox is fundamental to protecting the health of children and the community in general. Raising awareness about the disease, its forms of transmission and the importance of vaccination are essential steps towards controlling and eventually eradicating chickenpox as a public health problem.

1.4 CLINICAL MANIFESTATIONS

Clinical manifestations usually begin with non-specific symptoms such as fever, tiredness, headache and loss of appetite. These initial symptoms usually last one to two days before the characteristic rash appears.

Chickenpox rashes are the most distinctive feature of the disease. They start as small red spots that quickly turn into fluid-filled blisters called vesicles. These vesicles can be very itchy. Over time, the blisters rupture, forming small sores that eventually turn into scabs. This cycle of rash development can occur in several waves, resulting in lesions at different stages of evolution at the same time.

On physical examination, in addition to the rash, fever and general malaise can be observed. The rash usually appears first on the face, trunk and scalp, and then spreads to the rest of the body. In some cases, lesions can also appear on the mucous membranes of the mouth, ears and eyelids. The number of lesions can vary from a few dozen to over 500, depending on the severity of the infection.

Chickenpox generally has a benign and self-limiting course, with most cases resolving within one to two weeks. However, it is important to monitor symptoms and lesions to avoid complications. One of the most common complications is secondary bacterial infection of the skin lesions, which can occur when children scratch the vesicles, introducing bacteria.

Other more serious complications, although rare, include pneumonia, encephalitis (inflammation of the brain), and Reye's syndrome, a serious condition that affects the liver and brain, especially if the child was treated with aspirin during the infection. People with compromised immune systems, newborns and pregnant women are more susceptible to developing severe complications.

1.5 DIAGNOSIS

The diagnosis of chickenpox is usually clinical, i.e. based on the symptoms and characteristics of the rash. The observation of fluid-filled blisters that turn into scabs is quite characteristic and helps doctors to identify the disease easily. In addition, the presence of fever and other symptoms such as tiredness and loss of appetite also contribute to the diagnosis.

In cases where the diagnosis is not clear just by observing the symptoms and lesions, some laboratory tests can be carried out to confirm chickenpox. One of the most common tests is to detect specific antibodies against the varicella-zoster virus in the blood. This test can show whether the person has recently been infected by the virus.

Another useful test is the PCR (polymerase chain reaction) test, which detects the DNA of the varicella-zoster virus in skin lesions. This test is very accurate and can confirm the presence of the virus even in cases where the lesions are not typical or when the patient has a compromised immune system, making clinical identification difficult.

In addition, in specific situations, such as in patients with severe symptoms or complications, it may be necessary to carry out additional tests to assess the general state of health and identify possible complications. These tests may include chest X-rays to check for pneumonia and neurological tests if there is a suspicion of central nervous system involvement, such as encephalitis.

However, in most cases, chickenpox is diagnosed based on the clinical signs and symptoms observed by the doctor. It is important to consult a health professional at the first sign of chickenpox to confirm the diagnosis and receive advice on managing the disease, as well as preventing possible complications and transmission to other people.

1.6 TREATMENT

The treatment of chickenpox is mainly focused on relieving the symptoms, as the disease usually resolves on its own within one to two weeks. To control fever, the use of antipyretics such as paracetamol is recommended. The use of aspirin in children with chickenpox should be avoided, as it is associated with Reye's syndrome, a rare but serious condition that affects the liver and brain.

To relieve the itching caused by rashes, you can use calamine-based soothing lotions or take warm baths with colloidal oatmeal. These measures help to soothe the skin and reduce discomfort. It is important to keep children's nails trimmed and clean to prevent them from scratching the blisters and causing secondary infections. In cases of intense itching, the doctor may prescribe antihistamines to relieve the symptoms.

In the most severe cases, especially in patients with a compromised immune system, the doctor may recommend antiviral drugs such as acyclovir. These drugs help to reduce the severity and duration of the disease, as well as preventing complications. However, antivirals are generally reserved for people who are at greater risk of serious complications.

Prevention of chickenpox is possible and highly recommended through vaccination. The chickenpox vaccine is effective in preventing the disease and its complications. It is usually administered in two doses: the first at 12-15 months of age and the second between 4 and 6 years. Vaccination not only protects the individual, but also helps to reduce the spread of the virus in the community. Even if a vaccinated person does contract chickenpox, the symptoms will generally be milder and the recovery faster. In addition to vaccination, other preventive measures include avoiding contact with infected people and maintaining good hygiene practices, such as frequent hand washing.

1.7 PROGNOSIS

The prognosis for chickenpox is generally good, especially in healthy people with no complications. Most patients recover completely from the disease within one to two weeks, without permanent sequelae. However, in some cases, especially in people with weakened immune systems, newborns and pregnant women, chickenpox can lead to serious complications such as pneumonia, encephalitis and secondary skin infections.

The prevention of complications and a good prognosis depend on proper diagnosis and management of the disease. It is important to seek medical advice at the first sign of chickenpox and to follow the health professional's recommendations. In addition, vaccination against chickenpox is highly recommended to protect against the disease and its complications, thus reducing the risk of serious complications and improving patients' prognosis.

CHAPTER 2. RUBELLA

2.1 DEFINITION

Rubella is a contagious viral disease, also known as German measles. It is caused by the rubella virus (RV), which belongs to the Togaviridae family. The disease is usually mild in children, but can be more serious in adults, especially pregnant women, as it poses a risk to the fetus.

The history of rubella goes back centuries, but it wasn't until 1814 that the disease was first described. However, the causative virus was only identified in 1962, which made it possible to develop vaccines to prevent infection. Before then, rubella was a common disease, especially in children, but it caused concern due to the risk of complications in pregnant women.

The general characteristics of rubella include a low-grade fever, swollen lymph nodes and a red rash that usually starts on the face and spreads to the rest of the body. The rash tends to last around three days and is often accompanied by cold-like symptoms. The disease is highly contagious and can spread easily from one person to another through direct contact with respiratory secretions from infected people.

The etiological agent of rubella, the rubella virus (RV), is transmitted mainly through the air, when an infected person coughs or sneezes, releasing droplets containing the virus. The incubation period for rubella is usually 14 to 21 days, which means that a person can be infected and transmit the virus even before showing symptoms. This makes the prevention of rubella through vaccination an important measure to avoid the spread of the disease.

2.2 EPIDEMIOLOGY

Rubella was once a common disease in many parts of the world, but due to the effectiveness of vaccination, cases have decreased significantly. Before the introduction of the rubella vaccine, the disease was more prevalent in children and young adults. However, with large-scale vaccination programs, the incidence of rubella has fallen dramatically in many countries.

In Brazil, vaccination against rubella began in 1992, as part of the triple viral vaccine, which protects against measles, mumps and rubella. Since then, cases of rubella in the country have fallen considerably. In 2015, Brazil received the rubella elimination certificate from the Pan American Health Organization (PAHO), which means that there have been no autochthonous cases of the disease for at least three consecutive years.

However, it is important to maintain surveillance and vaccination coverage to ensure that rubella remains a controlled disease. Vaccination is the best way to prevent rubella and its complications, protecting not only the vaccinated individual, but also contributing to collective immunity and the protection of the entire community. Therefore, raising awareness about the importance of vaccination and easy access to vaccines are fundamental to maintaining the eradication of rubella and guaranteeing public health.

2.3 PHYSIOPATHOLOGY

When a person is infected with the virus, it multiplies in the cells of the upper respiratory tract and spreads through the body via the bloodstream. The virus can be transmitted through contact with an infected person's respiratory secretions, such as droplets of saliva or mucus, when coughing or sneezing.

The incubation period for rubella, i.e. the time between exposure to the virus and the appearance of symptoms, is usually between 14 and 21 days. During this period, the infected person can transmit the virus even before showing symptoms. Rubella is most contagious around a week before and a week after the appearance of the rash.

The clinical manifestations of rubella include a low-grade fever, swollen lymph nodes and a red rash that usually starts on the face and spreads to the rest of the body. The rash lasts two to three days and is often accompanied by cold-like symptoms such as a runny nose and cough. Most people recover completely from rubella without serious complications, but in rare cases, especially in pregnant women, the disease can lead to more serious complications.

Rubella can be prevented by vaccination. The rubella vaccine is usually administered as part of the triple viral vaccine, which also protects against measles and mumps. Vaccination is highly effective in preventing rubella and its complications. In addition to vaccination, simple hygiene measures, such as washing hands frequently and avoiding close contact with infected people, also help prevent the spread of the virus. It is important that people understand the importance of vaccination in order to protect not only themselves, but also the community as a whole.

2.4 CLINICAL MANIFESTATIONS

The most common symptoms of rubella include a low-grade fever, swollen lymph nodes and a red rash that starts on the face and spreads over the body. The rash usually lasts two to three days and can be accompanied by cold-like symptoms such as a runny nose and cough.

When examining a person with suspected rubella, the doctor can observe the typical signs of the disease. This includes the presence of a red rash, which is usually the main finding on physical examination. In addition, the lymph nodes, especially those in the neck and behind the ears, may be swollen and tender to the touch.

In most cases, rubella has a benign and self-limiting course, with symptoms disappearing within one to two weeks. However, in rare cases, especially in pregnant women, the disease can lead to more serious complications. One of the most worrying complications of rubella is congenital rubella syndrome, which occurs when the mother is infected during pregnancy and the virus affects the fetus. This can lead to serious birth defects, including deafness, heart problems, blindness and developmental delay.

Other less common complications of rubella include encephalitis, an inflammation of the brain, and thrombocytopenia, a decrease in the number of platelets in the blood. Although these complications are rare, it is important to be aware of them and seek medical attention if worrying symptoms arise during the rubella infection.

2.5 DIAGNOSIS

The diagnosis of rubella is usually made on the basis of the symptoms and the physical examination carried out by the doctor. The main signs of the disease include a low-grade fever, swollen lymph nodes and a red rash that starts on the face and spreads down the body. When examining the patient, the doctor can observe the presence of the rash and check whether the lymph nodes are enlarged and sensitive to touch.

In addition to the clinical examination, blood tests can be carried out to confirm the diagnosis of rubella. One of the most common tests is a test to detect specific antibodies against the rubella virus. This test can show whether the person has recently been infected by the virus. Another test that can be carried out is PCR (polymerase chain reaction), which detects the DNA of the rubella virus in blood samples.

In some cases, when there are doubts about the diagnosis or suspicions of complications, the doctor may order other complementary tests, such as a biopsy of the swollen lymph nodes or imaging tests, such as chest X-rays. These tests help to assess the patient's state of health and rule out other diseases with similar symptoms.

It is important to see a doctor at the first sign of rubella so that the diagnosis can be made correctly and appropriate treatment can be started, if necessary. In addition, confirmation of the diagnosis is important to avoid spreading the disease to other people and to prevent serious complications, especially in pregnant women.

2.6 TREATMENT

Treatment for rubella is generally aimed at relieving symptoms and preventing complications. As rubella is caused by a virus, antibiotics are not effective in treating the disease. Instead, the main focus is on providing supportive care to help the body fight the infection.

To relieve fever and discomfort, antipyretic drugs such as paracetamol can be used, according to medical advice. These drugs help to reduce fever and relieve mild pain associated with the illness. It is important to follow the doctor's instructions or the instructions on the label when taking any medication.

In addition to symptomatic treatment, rubella prevention is essential to prevent the spread of the disease and protect people at risk, especially pregnant women. The best way to prevent rubella is through vaccination. The rubella vaccine is usually administered as part of the triple viral vaccine, which also protects against measles and mumps. This vaccine is highly effective in preventing infection with the rubella virus and its complications.

Maintaining good hygiene practices, such as washing hands regularly and avoiding close contact with infected people, can also help prevent the spread of rubella. In addition, it is important that people are aware of the symptoms of rubella and seek medical attention at the first sign of the disease, so that the diagnosis can be made correctly and preventative measures can be taken to avoid the spread of the disease.

2.7 PROGNOSIS

The prognosis for rubella patients is generally good, especially in mild cases and in healthy people. In most cases, rubella resolves on its own in about one to two weeks, without leaving permanent sequelae. However, in rare cases, especially in pregnant women, rubella can lead to more serious complications, such as congenital rubella syndrome, which affects the development of the fetus and can cause serious birth defects.

To ensure a favorable prognosis and prevent complications, it is important that rubella patients receive proper care and follow medical guidelines. In addition, preventing rubella through vaccination is fundamental to avoiding infection and protecting the health of the community as a whole. Knowing the symptoms of rubella and seeking early medical attention can ensure a safe and speedy recovery.

CHAPTER 3. SUDDEN EXANTHEMA

3.1 DEFINITION

Sudden exanthema, also known as roseola infantum, is a viral disease common in young children, usually under 2 years of age. The term "exanthem" refers to a rash, while "sudden" indicates that the rash appears quickly after the onset of fever. This disease is mainly caused by human herpes virus type 6 (HHV-6), although human herpes virus type 7 (HHV-7) can also play a role in some cases.

The history of rash goes back many decades, but it was only in the middle of the 20th century that the human herpes virus type 6 was identified as the main causative agent of the disease. Sudden exanthema is a common childhood illness that is generally benign and self-limiting. Its general characteristics include the abrupt onset of a high fever, which lasts three to five days, followed by the sudden appearance of a pink rash, which usually starts on the trunk and spreads to other parts of the body.

3.2 EPIDEMIOLOGY

Sudden exanthema is a common childhood illness, mainly affecting children between the ages of 6 months and 2 years. It is found all over the world and occurs all year round, with no specific seasonality. Although it is a common viral illness, it is difficult to accurately estimate its prevalence and incidence, as many cases can go unnoticed or be misdiagnosed as other febrile illnesses in young children. In Brazil, as in other countries, exanthema súbito is a common childhood illness, but many cases may go unnoticed due to its self-limiting nature and mild symptoms.

3.3 PHYSIOPATHOLOGY

Sudden exanthema is caused by the human herpes virus type 6 (HHV-6) and, in some cases, the human herpes virus type 7 (HHV-7). These viruses are transmitted from person to person through contact with respiratory droplets or infected saliva. After infection, the virus replicates in the cells of the upper respiratory tract and spreads to other parts of the body, causing fever and other symptoms.

The rash infection cycle begins with the incubation period, which is the time between exposure to the virus and the onset of symptoms. This is followed by the sudden appearance of a pink rash, which starts on the trunk and spreads to other parts of the body. Most cases of rash are benign and resolve on their own within a few days, without complications.

To prevent the transmission of rash, it's important to practice hygiene measures, such as washing your hands frequently and avoiding close contact with infected people. However, as the disease is common in childhood and many cases go unnoticed, there is no effective way to prevent infection altogether. Vaccination against HHV-6 and HHV-7 is not yet available, but most children develop immunity after the initial infection.

3.4 CLINICAL MANIFESTATIONS

Sudden exanthema is characterized by a high fever followed by the abrupt appearance of a pink rash. Fever is usually the first symptom and can last from three to five days. Once the fever is gone, the rash appears, which is made up of small pink or red spots. These spots usually start on the trunk and spread to other parts of the body, such as the neck, arms and legs.

When examining a child with suspected rash, the doctor may notice the presence of the characteristic rash. In addition, enlarged lymph nodes can be found in some children. Other common signs and symptoms include irritability, lack of appetite and mild cold symptoms such as a runny nose and cough.

The course of the rash is generally benign and self-limiting. The fever disappears spontaneously after a few days and the rash tends to disappear in around one to three days, without leaving permanent sequelae. In most cases, there are no serious complications associated with the rash. However, in rare cases, the high fever can lead to febrile convulsions, especially in younger children.

It is important that parents are aware of the signs and symptoms of rash and seek medical attention if their child has a high fever or an unusual rash. Although most cases are benign and resolve on their own, it is important to rule out other causes of fever and rash, especially in children under 2 years of age.

3.5 DIAGNOSIS

The diagnosis of rash is usually made on the basis of the characteristic symptoms of the disease, such as a high fever followed by the appearance of a pink rash. The doctor may carry out a physical examination to observe the rash and check for other associated signs, such as enlarged lymph nodes. There are no specific tests to diagnose rash, as the disease is usually recognized clinically based on the typical symptoms presented by the child.

In some cases, the doctor may order blood tests to rule out other causes of fever and rash, especially if the symptoms are severe or persistent. However, these tests are generally not necessary to confirm the diagnosis of rash. The diagnosis is mainly based on the clinical history and the findings of the physical examination carried out by the doctor. If there is any doubt about the diagnosis or if the symptoms persist, the doctor may refer the child to a specialist for further evaluation.

3.6 TREATMENT

There is no specific treatment for rash, as the disease usually resolves on its own within a few days. Treatment aims to relieve symptoms such as fever and discomfort while the body fights the virus. This can include the use of antipyretic drugs, such as paracetamol, to reduce fever and relieve discomfort. It is important to follow the doctor's instructions or the medicine label when taking any medication.

As for the prevention of rash, there is no specific vaccine available to prevent infection with human herpes virus type 6 (HHV-6) or human herpes virus type 7 (HHV-7), which are the main causative agents of the disease. However, simple hygiene measures, such as washing your hands regularly and avoiding close contact with infected people, can help reduce the risk of contracting the virus. In addition, it is important to be aware of the signs and symptoms of rash and seek medical attention if a high fever or an unusual rash occurs, especially in young children.

3.7 PROGNOSIS

The prognosis for patients with rash is generally excellent, as the disease is self-limiting and benign in most cases. The high fever usually subsides within a few days, followed by the disappearance of the pink rash in around one to three days. In most cases, there are no serious complications associated with the rash, and recovery is complete. However, in rare cases, the high fever can lead to febrile convulsions, especially in younger children. It is important to seek medical attention if severe or persistent symptoms occur, to ensure proper management and rule out other conditions.

CHAPTER 4. INFECTIOUS ERYTHEMA

4.1 DEFINITION

Erythema infectiosum, also known as fifth disease or parvovirus, is a common viral disease that mainly affects school-age children, but can also occur in adults. It is caused by parvovirus B19, a virus that infects and destroys red blood cell precursor cells in the bone marrow. The name "erythema infectiosum" derives from the reddish rash that appears on the cheeks, similar to a slap on the face, which is a striking feature of the disease.

The history of erythema infectiosum goes back many years, but it was only in 1975 that parvovirus B19 was identified as the etiological agent responsible for the disease. Erythema infectiosum is highly contagious and is transmitted from person to person through direct contact with infected respiratory secretions, such as droplets of saliva or mucus. The disease is most common during the winter and spring months, and many outbreaks occur in school and nursery environments.

4.2 EPIDEMIOLOGY

Erythema infectiosum is a common disease worldwide, mainly affecting school-age children. The prevalence of the disease varies according to region and socio-economic conditions, but generally occurs in seasonal outbreaks during the winter and spring months. In Brazil, erythema infectiosum is also a common disease, especially in urban and densely populated areas, where contact between people is more frequent. Despite being a contagious disease, most infected people recover completely without serious complications.

4.3 PHYSIOPATHOLOGY

The pathophysiology of erythema infectiosum begins when the parvovirus B19 enters the human body, usually via the respiratory tract. After infection, the virus replicates and spreads to other parts of the body, including the bone marrow, where it infects and destroys the precursor cells of red blood cells. This can lead to a temporary decrease in red blood cell production, causing anemia in some cases.

Erythema infectiosum is transmitted through direct contact with infected respiratory secretions, such as droplets of saliva or mucus from an infected person. The virus can also be transmitted through contact with objects or surfaces contaminated by the virus. The disease cycle begins with the incubation period, which usually lasts between 4 and 14 days, followed by the appearance of the first symptoms, such as fever, headache and runny nose. After a few days, the characteristic rash may appear on the cheeks, followed by a red rash on the extremities of the body.

There is no vaccine available to prevent erythema infectiosum, but simple hygiene measures can help reduce the risk of infection. This includes washing hands regularly with soap and water, avoiding close contact with infected people and covering the mouth and nose when coughing or sneezing. It is important that people stay at home and avoid contact with other people while they are ill to prevent the spread of the virus. Most cases of erythema infectiosum are mild and resolve on their own, without specific treatment. However, in rare cases, serious complications can occur, especially in people with compromised immune systems.

4.4 CLINICAL MANIFESTATIONS

Erythema infectiosum has several distinct clinical manifestations. The first sign is often a low-grade fever, followed by symptoms such as headache, sore throat and tiredness. After a few days, a characteristic rash can occur, which usually starts on the cheeks, giving the appearance of "slapped cheeks". This rash can spread to the trunk and extremities of the body.

When examining a person with suspected erythema infectiosum, the doctor may notice the presence of the typical rash on the cheeks and possibly other areas of the body. In addition, the lymph nodes may be enlarged in some people. The course of erythema infectiosum is usually benign and self-limiting. The fever and initial symptoms usually subside in about a week, while the rash can persist for several weeks before disappearing completely.

In most cases, erythema infectiosum does not cause significant complications and recovery is complete. However, in some people, especially those with compromised immune systems, more serious complications can occur. One of the most common complications is viral arthritis, which causes pain and inflammation in the joints. In rare cases, erythema infectiosum can also lead to more serious complications, such as aplastic anemia, which is a decrease in the production of red blood cells in the bone marrow. It is important to seek medical attention if severe or persistent symptoms occur.

4.5 DIAGNOSIS

The diagnosis of erythema infectiosum is usually made on the basis of the characteristic symptoms of the disease, such as fever and a rash on the cheeks. The doctor may carry out a physical examination to observe the rash and check for other associated signs, such as enlarged lymph nodes. There are no specific tests to diagnose erythema infectiosum, as the disease is usually recognized clinically based on the typical symptoms presented by the person.

In some cases, the doctor may order blood tests to confirm the diagnosis of erythema infectiosum or rule out other conditions. These tests may include testing for antibodies against parvovirus B19 or detecting the virus itself in the blood. However, these tests are generally not necessary to confirm the diagnosis, unless there are doubts about the cause of the illness. It is important to consult a doctor if you or your child experience symptoms of erythema infectiosum in order to obtain an accurate diagnosis and appropriate treatment guidelines.

4.6 TREATMENT

There is no specific treatment for erythema infectiosum, as the disease usually resolves on its own without serious complications. Treatment is mainly aimed at relieving symptoms such as fever and discomfort. This can include the use of antipyretic drugs, such as paracetamol, to reduce fever and relieve pain. It is important to follow medical advice when taking any medication and to ensure adequate hydration by drinking plenty of fluids.

As for preventing erythema infectiosum, simple hygiene measures can help reduce the risk of infection. This includes washing your hands regularly with soap and water, especially after coughing, sneezing or blowing your nose. In addition, it is important to avoid close contact with infected people and to cover your mouth and nose when coughing or sneezing. There is no vaccine available to prevent erythema infectiosum, but following these hygiene practices can help reduce the risk of infection and the spread of the virus. If you or your child experience symptoms of erythema infectiosum, it is important to consult a doctor for specific treatment and care guidelines.

4.7 PROGNOSIS

The prognosis for patients with erythema infectiosum is generally excellent, as most cases are mild and resolve on their own without serious complications. The fever and characteristic rash tend to disappear within a few weeks, and recovery is complete. However, in some rare cases,

especially in people with compromised immune systems, more serious complications can occur, such as viral arthritis or aplastic anemia. It is important to seek medical attention if severe or persistent symptoms occur, to ensure proper management and avoid complications.

CHAPTER 5. SCARLET FEVER

5.1 DEFINITION

Scarlet fever is a bacterial infection caused by the bacterium Streptococcus pyogenes, also known as group A streptococcus. This disease can affect people of all ages, but is most common in children between the ages of 5 and 15. It is characterized by a red rash that can resemble the texture of sandpaper, especially in the folds of the skin, such as the armpits, groin and neck.

Historically, scarlet fever was a much more common and serious disease before the advent of antibiotics. In the 19th century, it was one of the main causes of infant mortality. However, with the widespread use of antibiotics to treat streptococcal infections, the incidence and severity of scarlet fever decreased significantly. Today, the disease is considered less common and, in most cases, is treatable with effective antibiotics.

5.2 EPIDEMIOLOGY

Scarlet fever is a disease that occurs all over the world, but its incidence varies according to factors such as geographical region, socio-economic conditions and access to health care. In areas where people are more crowded, such as schools and nurseries, transmission of the Streptococcus pyogenes bacteria responsible for scarlet fever can be more common. In Brazil, scarlet fever is still present, although less frequently than in the past, due to advances in public health and the use of antibiotics to treat streptococcal infections.

The incidence of scarlet fever can be seasonal, with an increase in cases during the colder months of the year. This may be related to a greater likelihood of the bacteria spreading indoors and in crowded environments during the winter. Although scarlet fever can occur in people of all ages, it is most common in children between the ages of 5 and 15. It is important to seek medical attention if scarlet fever is suspected, so that the correct diagnosis can be made and appropriate treatment started as soon as possible.

5.3 PHYSIOPATHOLOGY

Scarlet fever is caused by the bacterium Streptococcus pyogenes, which is also known as group A streptococcus. This bacterium produces toxins that cause the characteristic symptoms of the disease. When a person is infected with Streptococcus pyogenes, the toxins released by the bacteria can trigger an inflammatory response in the body, resulting in symptoms such as fever, sore throat and rash.

The transmission of scarlet fever occurs mainly through direct contact with respiratory droplets from an infected person. This can happen when talking, coughing or sneezing. The bacteria can also be transmitted through contact with contaminated objects, such as toys or utensils. Once inside the body, Streptococcus pyogenes can multiply rapidly and cause infection. To prevent scarlet fever, it is important to practice good hygiene, such as washing your hands regularly and avoiding close contact with infected people. Early treatment with antibiotics is also essential to prevent complications and stop the spread of the disease.

5.4 CLINICAL MANIFESTATIONS

Scarlet fever is known for having a characteristic rash that starts on the neck and chest and spreads to the rest of the body. This rash usually resembles "sandpaper skin", with red, raised spots that can be painful to the touch. In addition to the rash, other common symptoms include high fever, sore throat, general malaise, headache and enlarged lymph nodes in the neck.

When examining a person with suspected scarlet fever, the doctor may notice the presence of the characteristic rash, especially in the neck and chest areas. In addition, signs of pharyngitis may be found, such as redness and swelling in the throat. Sometimes the tongue can become covered in a white substance with red spots, giving the appearance of a "raspberry tongue". In severe or complicated cases, scarlet fever can lead to complications such as rheumatic fever, acute glomerulonephritis, peritonsillar abscesses or pneumonia.

Most cases of scarlet fever are mild and resolve on their own with appropriate treatment. The use of antibiotics, such as penicillin or amoxicillin, is common to treat the bacterial infection caused by Streptococcus pyogenes and help prevent complications. With proper treatment, symptoms usually improve within a week. However, it is important to follow the doctor's instructions and complete the full course of antibiotics prescribed, even if symptoms improve sooner. In severe or complicated cases, hospitalization and additional treatment may be required to manage complications.

5.5 DIAGNOSIS

The diagnosis of scarlet fever is usually based on the characteristic symptoms presented by the patient, such as high fever, sore throat and a rash that resembles "sandpaper skin". The doctor may also examine the throat for signs of streptococcal pharyngitis, such as redness and swelling. There is no specific test to diagnose scarlet fever, but in some cases, the doctor may carry out a throat culture test to confirm the presence of Streptococcus pyogenes bacteria.

The throat culture test involves taking a sample of throat secretion and culturing it in the laboratory to detect the presence of Streptococcus pyogenes bacteria. In addition, a rapid streptococcal antigen test can be carried out to quickly detect the presence of the bacteria within minutes. However, it is important to remember that these tests may not be necessary in all cases of scarlet fever and that the diagnosis is usually made on the basis of the symptoms and the physical examination carried out by the doctor. If you or your child experience symptoms of scarlet fever, it is important to consult a doctor for an accurate diagnosis and appropriate treatment guidelines.

5.6 TREATMENT

Treatment for scarlet fever usually involves the use of antibiotics to fight the bacterial infection caused by the bacterium Streptococcus pyogenes. The most commonly prescribed antibiotics include penicillin and amoxicillin, which are effective against this bacterium. It is important to follow the doctor's instructions and complete the full course of antibiotics prescribed, even if symptoms improve earlier. This helps to ensure complete elimination of the bacteria and reduces the risk of complications.

To prevent scarlet fever, it's important to practice good hygiene, such as washing your hands regularly with soap and water, especially after coughing, sneezing or blowing your nose. It is also important to avoid close contact with infected people and to cover your mouth and nose when coughing or sneezing. There is no vaccine available to prevent scarlet fever, but following these hygiene practices can help reduce the risk of infection and the spread of the virus. If you or your child experience symptoms of scarlet fever, it is important to consult a doctor for specific treatment and care guidelines.

5.7 PROGNOSIS

The prognosis for scarlet fever patients is generally excellent, especially when the disease is diagnosed early and treated properly with antibiotics. Most cases of scarlet fever are mild and resolve on their own with appropriate treatment. With antibiotics, symptoms usually improve in about a week. Serious complications are rare, especially in healthy people, but can occur in rare cases, such as rheumatic fever or acute glomerulonephritis. It is important to follow the doctor's instructions and complete the full course of antibiotics prescribed to ensure a full recovery and avoid complications.

CHAPTER 6. MEASLES

6.1 DEFINITION

Measles is an infectious disease caused by the Measles virus, which is highly contagious. The virus spreads easily through direct contact with an infected person's respiratory secretions, such as sneezing or coughing. After exposure to the virus, symptoms usually appear within 10 to 14 days.

Measles was a common and often fatal disease before the introduction of the measles vaccine. However, thanks to vaccination efforts around the world, the number of cases has dropped significantly. Symptoms of measles include fever, cough, runny nose, red and light-sensitive eyes, and a characteristic rash that starts on the face and spreads down the body. Although most people recover completely, measles can cause serious complications, especially in young children, the elderly and people with compromised immune systems.

6.2 EPIDEMIOLOGY

Measles is a highly contagious disease that affects people of all ages and occurs all over the world. Before the introduction of the measles vaccine, the disease was very common and caused devastating epidemics. However, thanks to vaccination efforts in many countries, the incidence of measles has decreased significantly in recent decades.

In Brazil, measles is still a public health concern, although mass vaccination has reduced the number of cases. However, occasional outbreaks still occur, especially in areas where vaccination coverage is low. It is important to ensure that everyone receives the necessary doses of the measles vaccine to prevent the spread of the disease.

Vaccination is the main way of preventing measles. The triple viral vaccine, which protects against measles, mumps and rubella, is highly effective and is usually administered in two doses during childhood. Maintaining high vaccination rates is key to preventing outbreaks and protecting communities against measles. In addition, infection control measures, such as washing hands regularly and avoiding close contact with infected people, are also important to prevent the spread of the virus.

6.3 PHYSIOPATHOLOGY

Measles is caused by the measles virus and spreads easily from person to person through direct contact with respiratory droplets from an infected person. The virus can remain in the air and on surfaces for up to two hours, making transmission very effective. After exposure to the virus, it replicates in the cells of the respiratory tract and spreads throughout the body via the lymphatic system and the blood.

The symptoms of measles usually appear around 10 to 14 days after exposure to the virus and include fever, cough, runny nose, red and light-sensitive eyes, and a characteristic rash that spreads from the face to the rest of the body. The best way to prevent measles is through vaccination. The triple viral vaccine, which protects against measles, mumps and rubella, is highly effective and is usually administered in two doses during childhood. Maintaining high vaccination rates is key to preventing outbreaks and protecting communities against measles. In addition, infection control measures, such as washing hands regularly and avoiding close contact with infected people, are also important to prevent the spread of the virus.

6.4 CLINICAL MANIFESTATIONS

The clinical manifestations of measles usually begin with cold-like symptoms such as fever, cough, runny nose and red, light-sensitive eyes. After a few days, a characteristic rash appears, starting on the face and spreading over the body. This rash consists of flat red spots that merge and can become raised.

When examining a patient with suspected measles, the doctor may notice the presence of the characteristic rash, especially in the face and neck areas. In addition, signs of pharyngitis may be found, such as redness and swelling in the throat. In severe cases, the patient may develop complications such as pneumonia, encephalitis (inflammation of the brain) and otitis media (middle ear infection).

Most cases of measles resolve on their own, but there can be serious complications, especially in young children, the elderly and people with compromised immune systems. It is important to seek medical attention if measles is suspected, so that the correct diagnosis can be made and appropriate treatment started as soon as possible. In severe cases, hospitalization and treatment to manage complications may be necessary.

6.5 DIAGNOSIS

The diagnosis of measles is usually based on the symptoms presented by the patient and their history of exposure to the virus. The doctor may carry out a physical examination to check for the presence of the characteristic rash and other signs of the disease, such as fever and cough. In addition, the doctor may ask about the patient's recent travel history and vaccination history.

In some cases, a blood test may be carried out to confirm the diagnosis of measles. This test can detect the presence of antibodies against the measles virus in the patient's blood. In addition, a sample of nasal or throat secretions can be taken and sent to a laboratory for specific tests to detect the virus. However, the diagnosis of measles is usually made on the basis of the symptoms and the physical examination carried out by the doctor. If you or your child show symptoms of measles, it is important to consult a doctor for an accurate diagnosis and appropriate treatment guidelines.

6.6 TREATMENT

There is no specific treatment for measles, but the symptoms can be managed to help the patient feel better while the body fights the infection. This can include rest, adequate hydration and the use of medication for fever and discomfort, such as paracetamol. In some cases, hospitalization may be necessary, especially if there are serious complications.

The best way to prevent measles is through vaccination. The triple viral vaccine, which protects against measles, mumps and rubella, is highly effective and is usually administered in two doses during childhood. Maintaining high vaccination rates is key to preventing outbreaks and protecting communities against measles. In addition, infection control measures, such as washing hands regularly and avoiding close contact with infected people, are also important to prevent the spread of the virus.

6.7 PROGNOSIS

The prognosis for measles patients is generally good, especially when the disease is diagnosed and treated early. In most cases, the symptoms of measles disappear on their own in about one to two weeks. However, in some rare cases, measles can lead to serious complications, especially in young children, the elderly and people with compromised immune systems. Complications such as pneumonia, encephalitis (inflammation of the brain) and otitis media (middle ear infection) can occur, but are uncommon. It is important to seek medical attention if measles is suspected, so that the correct diagnosis can be made and appropriate treatment started as soon as possible, thus reducing the risk of complications.

CHAPTER 7. INFECTIOUS MONONUCLEOSIS

7.1 DEFINITION

Infectious mononucleosis, also known as "kissing disease" or "student kissing disease", is a common viral infection caused mainly by the Epstein-Barr virus (EBV). It usually affects teenagers and young adults and is transmitted mainly through saliva, close contact or sharing personal utensils such as glasses or cutlery. EBV is a virus from the Herpesviridae family and can remain in the body of an infected person for the rest of their life, although it usually remains inactive in most cases.

Infectious mononucleosis is characterized by flu-like symptoms such as fever, sore throat, extreme fatigue and enlarged lymph nodes. In addition, there is often an increase in the number of blood cells called lymphocytes, which are cells of the immune system. Complete recovery from infectious mononucleosis usually takes a few weeks to a few months, and symptoms can vary from mild to severe, depending on the person affected. In some rare cases, EBV infection can lead to more serious complications, such as inflammation of the liver (hepatitis), inflammation of the spleen (splenomegaly) or rupture of the spleen, especially if vigorous physical activity is involved during the acute phase of the disease.

7.2 EPIDEMIOLOGY

Infectious mononucleosis is a common disease worldwide, affecting mainly adolescents and young adults. The prevalence of the disease can vary according to factors such as age, lifestyle and geographical region. In Brazil, as in other countries, infectious mononucleosis is relatively common, especially among young people who attend schools, universities and community settings.

Infectious mononucleosis is usually transmitted through close contact with an infected person, mainly through saliva. This can happen when sharing personal utensils, such as glasses, cutlery or toothbrushes, or through kissing. As a result, the disease can spread rapidly in environments where people are in close proximity, such as schools and university dormitories. Although infectious mononucleosis is commonly associated with adolescence and youth, people of all ages can be affected by the disease.

7.3 PHYSIOPATHOLOGY

Infectious mononucleosis is mainly caused by the Epstein-Barr virus (EBV), which belongs to the Herpesviridae family. After exposure to EBV, the virus enters the body through the mucous membrane of the mouth and throat, where it infects cells of the immune system, such as B lymphocytes. The virus replicates within these cells and spreads throughout the body via the bloodstream.

Infectious mononucleosis is usually transmitted through close contact with an infected person, mainly through saliva. This can happen when sharing personal utensils, such as glasses, cutlery or toothbrushes, or through kissing. As a result, the disease can spread rapidly in environments where people are in close proximity, such as schools and university dormitories. Although infectious mononucleosis is commonly associated with adolescence and youth, people of all ages can be affected by the disease.

7.4 CLINICAL MANIFESTATIONS

The clinical manifestations of infectious mononucleosis usually include flu-like symptoms such as fever, sore throat, extreme fatigue and muscle aches. Other common symptoms include enlarged lymph nodes, especially in the neck and groin, and an enlarged liver and spleen, which can be detected during a physical examination.

When examining a patient with suspected infectious mononucleosis, the doctor can observe these physical signs, as well as checking for the presence of the characteristic rash, which can occur in some cases. The course of the disease varies from person to person, but generally symptoms begin to improve within a few weeks. However, extreme fatigue can persist for several weeks or months after the acute infection.

In some rare cases, infectious mononucleosis can lead to more serious complications, such as inflammation of the liver (hepatitis), inflammation of the spleen (splenomegaly) or rupture of the spleen. These complications are more common in adults than in children and may require additional treatment. It is important to seek medical attention if infectious mononucleosis is suspected, especially if there are signs of complications.

7.5 DIAGNOSIS

The diagnosis of infectious mononucleosis is usually based on the patient's symptoms, medical history and physical examination. The doctor may order blood tests to confirm the diagnosis, such as the heterophilia test, which checks for the presence of specific antibodies produced in response to infection by the Epstein-Barr virus (EBV). In addition, the doctor may perform a complete blood count to check for an increase in lymphocytes and the presence of other blood abnormalities associated with the disease.

Other imaging tests, such as abdominal ultrasound, can be carried out to assess the size and function of the liver and spleen, which are usually enlarged during acute infection. In some cases, a sample of tissue from the liver or spleen can be taken via a biopsy to confirm the diagnosis or rule out other conditions. It is important to consult a doctor if infectious mononucleosis is suspected, so that the correct diagnosis can be made and appropriate treatment started as soon as possible.

7.6 TREATMENT

There is no specific treatment for infectious mononucleosis, as it is a viral disease. Generally, treatment aims to relieve symptoms and promote patient comfort during the period of infection. This can include rest, drinking enough fluids to avoid dehydration and taking medication to relieve fever, sore throat and muscle pain. It is important to avoid drinking alcohol and taking medication that could overload the liver, as this organ may be compromised during the infection.

Prevention of infectious mononucleosis mainly involves measures to reduce the risk of exposure to the Epstein-Barr virus (EBV), which is the causative agent of the disease. This includes avoiding sharing personal utensils, such as glasses, cutlery and toothbrushes, and avoiding kissing infected people during the period when the disease is transmissible. In addition, washing your hands regularly with soap and water can help prevent the spread of the virus. There is no vaccine available to prevent infectious mononucleosis, but maintaining a healthy immune system through a balanced diet, regular exercise and adequate sleep can help reduce the risk of infection.

7.7 PROGNOSIS

The prognosis for patients with infectious mononucleosis is generally good, with most cases resolving on their own in a few weeks to a few months. Complete recovery is expected, but can take some time due to the prolonged fatigue that many patients experience. Serious complications are rare, but can occur, especially in adults. It is important to follow medical recommendations, get enough rest, stay hydrated and avoid strenuous activities during the infection period for a faster and more complete recovery.

CHAPTER 8. KAWASAKI DISEASE

8.1 DEFINITION

Kawasaki disease is an inflammatory disease that mainly affects young children, especially those under the age of five. It can cause inflammation in blood vessels throughout the body, including the coronary arteries that supply blood to the heart. Kawasaki disease is one of the main causes of acquired heart disease in children in developed countries, but its exact cause is still unknown.

Kawasaki disease was first described in 1967 by Japanese pediatrician Tomisaku Kawasaki. He identified a number of cases of children with similar symptoms, including persistent high fever, conjunctivitis, skin rash, swelling of the lymph nodes in the neck and inflammation of the blood vessels. Since then, the disease has been recognized worldwide. Its etiological agent is still not fully understood, but it is suspected to involve an abnormal immune system response to a viral or bacterial infection.

8.2 EPIDEMIOLOGY

Kawasaki disease is most common in children, especially between the ages of one and five. Although it can occur anywhere in the world, it is more prevalent in developed countries such as the United States and Japan. In Brazil, the incidence of the disease seems to be lower compared to other regions, but there are still cases reported throughout the country.

The incidence of Kawasaki disease varies according to factors such as age, gender and geographical location. It is not yet clear why some children develop the disease while others do not, but genetic and environmental factors may play an important role. Understanding the epidemiology of the disease is fundamental to developing effective prevention and treatment strategies.

8.3 PHYSIOPATHOLOGY

The pathophysiology of Kawasaki disease involves a generalized inflammatory response by the immune system, which affects blood vessels throughout the body. It is not yet clear what triggers this response, but it is believed that a viral or bacterial infection may be a triggering factor in genetically predisposed people. This inflammation can lead to the formation of aneurysms in the coronary arteries, which are blood vessels that supply the heart.

Kawasaki disease is not considered contagious, i.e. it is not transmitted from person to person. Instead, it is an autoimmune condition, which means that the person's own immune system mistakenly attacks healthy tissues in the body. The disease cycle can vary in each individual, but generally involves an acute phase of symptoms, followed by a sub-acute phase and finally a convalescent phase. The prevention of Kawasaki disease is not yet fully understood, but some studies suggest that exclusive breastfeeding in the first months of life can reduce the risk of developing the disease. In addition, it is important to maintain a healthy lifestyle, including a balanced diet and regular physical activity, to strengthen the immune system and reduce the risk of infections that can trigger the disease.

8.4 CLINICAL MANIFESTATIONS

The clinical manifestations of Kawasaki disease can vary in severity and can develop in phases over several weeks. Initial symptoms include persistent high fever for more than five days, irritability, conjunctivitis (red eyes), a rash all over the body, swelling of the hands and feet, as well as redness and peeling of the palms of the hands and soles of the feet. As the disease progresses, the symptoms can worsen and serious complications can occur, such as inflammation of the blood vessels (vasculitis) and aneurysms in the coronary arteries.

When examining a patient with suspected Kawasaki disease, the doctor can observe these physical signs, as well as checking for the presence of aneurysms in the coronary arteries, which can be detected using imaging tests such as echocardiography or magnetic resonance angiography (MRI). Early treatment is essential to reduce the risk of serious complications, such as coronary aneurysms, and can include the use of aspirin and intravenous immunoglobulin to reduce inflammation and prevent damage to blood vessels.

The course of Kawasaki disease varies from person to person, but most patients recover completely with appropriate treatment. However, some patients can develop serious complications, such as coronary aneurysms, which can increase the risk of long-term heart problems. That's why it's important to follow medical recommendations and carry out regular follow-ups to monitor heart health.

In rare cases, Kawasaki disease can lead to serious complications such as heart failure, cardiac arrhythmias and even death. It is therefore important to be aware of the warning signs and seek immediate medical attention if Kawasaki disease is suspected. With early diagnosis and treatment, many patients recover completely and have a good long-term quality of life.

8.5 DIAGNOSIS

The diagnosis of Kawasaki disease is mainly based on the symptoms presented by the patient and the exclusion of other conditions that could cause similar symptoms. There is no specific test to diagnose the disease, but the doctor may order a series of tests to help confirm the diagnosis. This can include blood tests to check the levels of inflammation in the body, such as C-reactive protein (CRP) and erythrocyte sedimentation rate (ESR).

In addition to blood tests, the doctor may also order an echocardiogram to check for abnormalities in the heart, such as aneurysms in the coronary arteries. This is an imaging test that uses sound waves to create an image of the heart and blood vessels. Other imaging tests, such as magnetic resonance angiography (MRA) or computed tomography (CT), can also be carried out to assess the state of the blood vessels. It is important to carry out these tests as soon as possible in order to start appropriate treatment and reduce the risk of serious complications.

8.6 TREATMENT

The treatment of Kawasaki disease usually involves the use of drugs to reduce inflammation and prevent complications. Two commonly used drugs are aspirin and intravenous immunoglobulin (IVIG). Aspirin is used in lower doses to help reduce fever and inflammation, while IVIG is administered to help decrease the immune system's inflammatory response.

In addition to drug treatment, rest and supportive care are also important during the recovery period. This includes ensuring that the child is getting enough rest, staying well hydrated and maintaining a healthy diet. In some cases, follow-up with pediatric cardiologists may be necessary to monitor heart health and detect any cardiac complications early on.

As for the prevention of Kawasaki disease, there is no specific way to prevent the disease from occurring, as its exact cause is still not fully understood. However, some studies suggest that exclusive breastfeeding in the first months of life may have a protective effect against the development of the disease. In addition, maintaining a healthy lifestyle, including a balanced diet, regular physical activity and hygiene measures such as frequent hand washing, can help strengthen the immune system and reduce the risk of infections that can trigger the disease.

8.7 PROGNOSIS

The prognosis for patients with Kawasaki disease is generally good, especially when treatment is started early. With proper treatment, most children recover completely from the disease without serious complications. However, in more severe cases or when treatment is not administered quickly, cardiac complications can occur, such as aneurysms in the coronary arteries, which can increase the risk of long-term heart problems. It is important to have regular medical follow-up to monitor heart health and ensure a full and healthy recovery.

REFERENCES

DE ALMEIDA PONTES, Cleuma Regina Freitas et al. Diagnostic Approach to Exanthematous Diseases in Childhood. **Brazilian Journal of Implantology and Health Sciences**, v. 6, n. 5, p. 623633, 2024.

DE AZEVEDO, Aida Correia et al. EXANTEMATIC DISEASES IN PEDIATRIC AGE - THEORETICAL REVIEW.

ELIDIO, Guilherme Almeida. Epidemiological situation of measles in Brazil in the post-elimination era: 2018 to 2019. 2023.

GARCIA, Kíssia Bárbara Sousa. The relevance of differential diagnosis in the clinical management of viral exanthematous diseases prevalent in childhood: a study on chickenpox, hand foot mouth, rubella and erythema infectiosum. 2023.

GILLI, Isadora Olenscki et al. ASYMETRIC PERIFLEXURAL EXANThem: DO YOU KNOW ABOUT THIS DISEASE? **Paranaense Journal of Pediatrics**, v. 22, n. 1, p. 1-3, 2021.

GONÇALVES, Angelina Maria Freire. Exanthematous diseases in childhood.

MENDONÇA, Dilton Rodrigues et al. MEDICINE INTEGRATED PRACTICES Teaching Plan 2023.1. 2023.

NOGUEIRA, Gabriela Fernandes et al. **Viral diseases in Brazil: emergencies and re-emergencies**. Editora Appris, 2021.

NUNES, Julianne Caixeta et al. Emerging exanthematous viral diseases with oral manifestations: measles and monkeypox. **Brazilian Journal of Implantology and Health Sciences**, v. 5, n. 4, p. 1407-1420, 2023.

SAKANE, Pedro Takanori et al. Common exanthematous diseases of childhood. In: **Laboratory medicine in pediatrics**. Manole, 2023.

SCHNEERSOHN, ABRAHAM NUNES CEZAR. EXANTHEMATOUS SYNDROMES.

SEGATTO, Teresa Cristina Vieira et al. Epidemiological profile of notified measles cases in the Federal District, 2009 to 2020. 2020.

SOARES, Claudia Regina Belo. DIAGNOSTIC APPROACH TO CHILDHOOD EXANTHEMATOUS DISEASES. **RCMOS-Revista Científica Multidisciplinar O Saber**, v. 1, n. 1, 2024.

UEDA, E. Y. K. et al. ERYTHROVIRUS B19 IN PEDIATRIC PATIENTS: A REVIEW OF THE LITERATURE. **Hematology, Transfusion and Cell Therapy**, v. 43, p. S285, 2021.

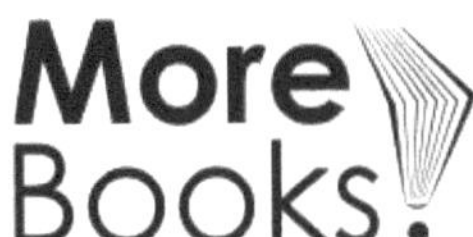

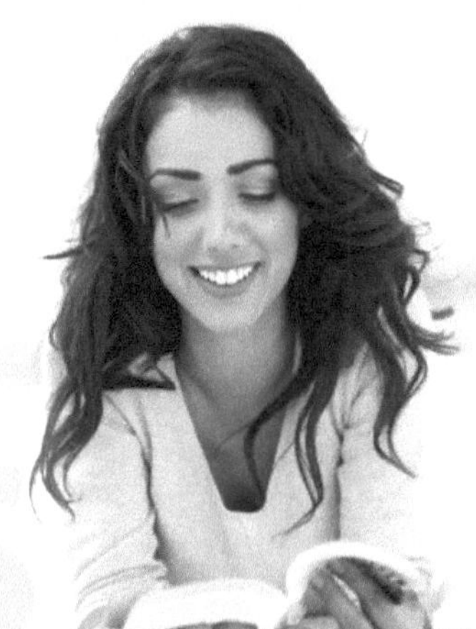

I want morebooks!

Buy your books fast and straightforward online - at one of world's fastest growing online book stores! Environmentally sound due to Print-on-Demand technologies.

Buy your books online at
www.morebooks.shop

Kaufen Sie Ihre Bücher schnell und unkompliziert online – auf einer der am schnellsten wachsenden Buchhandelsplattformen weltweit! Dank Print-On-Demand umwelt- und ressourcenschonend produziert.

Bücher schneller online kaufen
www.morebooks.shop

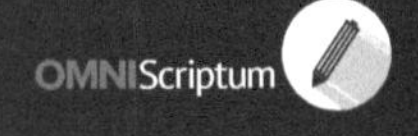

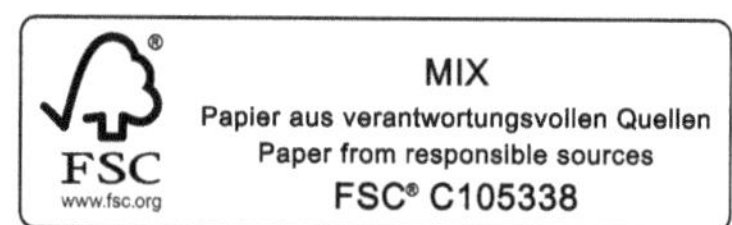

Printed by Books on Demand GmbH, Norderstedt / Germany